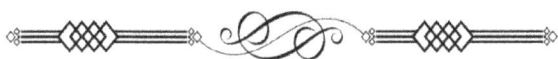

Church Nursing

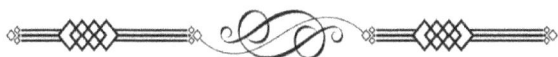

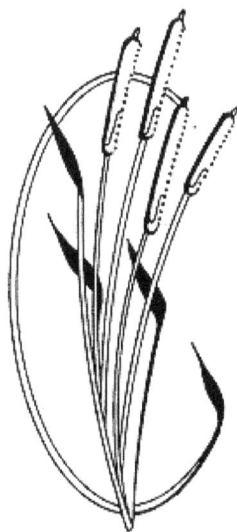

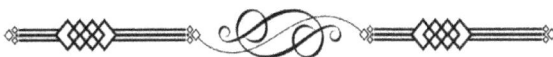

Church Nursing

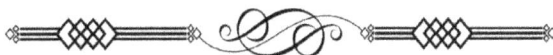

Dr. Juanita Crawford *Ed.D, MSN, RN*

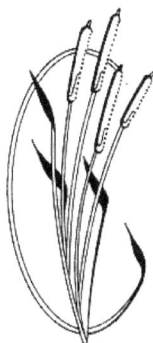

Senior Publisher
Steven Lawrence Hill Sr

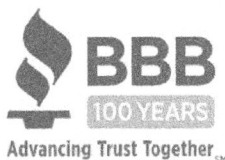

BBB
100 YEARS
Advancing Trust Together sm

A Publisher Trademark Title page

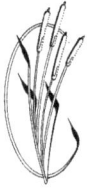

ASA Publishing Corporation
An Accredited Hybrid Publishing House with the BBB
www.asapublishingcorporation.com

The Landmark Building
23 E. Front St., Suite 103, Monroe, Michigan 48161

Copyrights©2018 Juanita Crawford, All Rights Reserved
Book Title: Church Nursing
Date Published: 05.18.2018 / Edition 1 *Trade Paperback*
Book ID: ASAPCID2380747
ISBN: 978-1-946746-31-3
Library of Congress Cataloging-in-Publication Data

This book was published in the United States of America.
Great State of Michigan

A Publisher Trademark Copyrights page

⁴¹ He who receives a prophet in the name of a prophet shall receive a prophet's reward. And he who receives a righteous man in the name of a righteous man shall receive a righteous man's reward. ⁴² And whoever gives one of these little ones only a cup of cold water in the name of a disciple, assuredly, I say to you, he shall by no means lose his reward."

St. Matthew 10:41-42
NKJV

FOREWORD

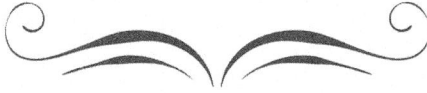

Have you ever had a desire to render service to the Lord by serving on an auxiliary in your church? Well, becoming a church nurse is very rewarding. Conversely, just as professional nursing, church nursing comes with challenges; and one must be alert, a critical thinker, and humbly ready to react.

As Christians we are held accountable for rendering services to the Glory of God and our conduct should exemplify doing things decently and in order (1st Corinthians 14:40, paraphrased). For God sees and hears all; we must be our best at all times, even when no one is watching. What a PRIVILEGE IT is to render services in the house of the lord; in particular, serving on the nurses' guild. May each individual reading this book who has a desire to be a church nurse OR who IS currently serving on a nurses' Guild or any other auxiliary, be blessed and edified.

DEDICATION

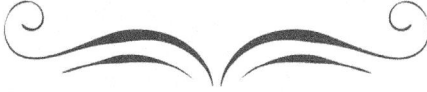

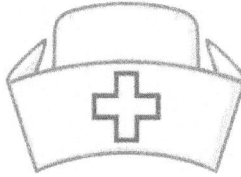

This book is dedicated to Church nurses all around the world who faithfully dedicate their services to the Lord, their Pastors, and church families. This book is dedicated to the nurses who in the past served under my leadership as President of the Nurse's Guild. This book is also dedicated to my dear sister (*Ms. Rebecca Johnson*) who serves faithfully on the nurses' guild (president) at one of my brother's church. May God continue to strengthen, guide, and edify you all throughout your careers, community services, and personal endeavors.

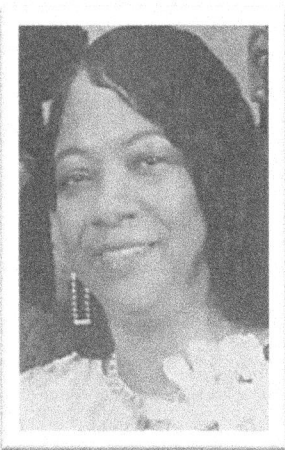

Ms. Rebecca Johnson

ACKNOWLEDGEMENTS

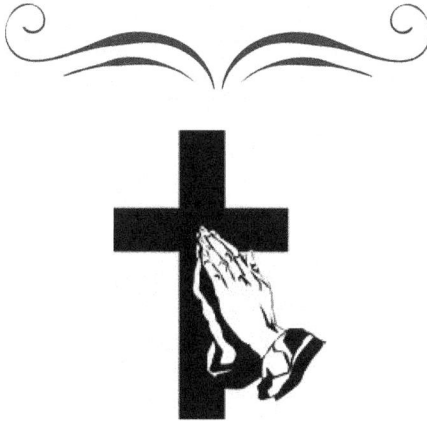

I give reverence to my Lord and Savior Jesus Christ for allowing me to write my 4th book. *Heavenly Father, I thank you for granting me patience, endurance, and continuity in writing to your Glory and all readers' edification.*

To my husband (Rev. Emmett Crawford Jr.), thank you for the initial phase of proof-reading and editing this book.

All Scriptures quoted and paraphrased are taken from the Holy Bible (KJV), unless otherwise denoted

Table of Contents

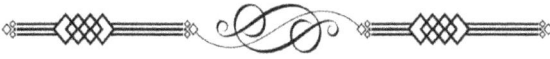

Church Nursing

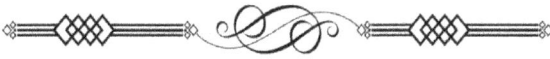

Dr. Juanita Crawford *Ed.D, MSN, RN*

CHAPTER 1
INTRODUCTION

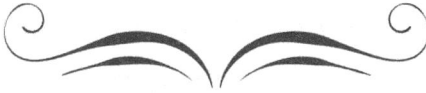

In my youth, serving the Lord and the profession as a nurse was one of my repetitive dreams, so in my mid-twenties the decision was made to become a church nurse; yet I didn't have a clue as to what I was supposed to be doing. While growing up in a Baptist church the only tasks I recall performed by the nurses on the guild was the serving of beverages to the pastor and the fanning of parishioners who appeared to have fainted. Even worst, after joining a nurses' guild at a past church I was lead into a room (Nurses' Guild on the door) by an older parishioner on the guild and informed to "just do what I tell you to do." All dressed in white (dress, hat, stockings, and shoes); the older parishioner then put me on a navy blue nursing cape. Wow, I felt good in my regalia, but I did nothing but sit on the pew. In fact, she served the pastor his beverage.

Well, this did not sit well with me.

After attending a new church I was asked to establish a nurses' guild. I accepted and begin to conduct research on church nursing; to my surprise only one book was available (that was decades ago) and to this day I cannot find that book. Thank God the book gave me the basics of church nursing, but since then trends in church nursing has evolved which prompted me to write this book. After serving on the nurses' guild for decades I decided to share with others who may be seeking information concerning nurses' guilds establishments in Baptist churches. I must say, my experience as a professional nurse assisted highly in the development of the guild and performing services as a church nurse. So what is the disparity between church nursing and professional nursing? Read on and you will find out, but I can say the congruence is "serving wholeheartedly, as if you were serving the Lord" (Ephesians 6:7). Respectfully, one must ascertain they want to be a church nurse, and because one is a professional nurse does not mean you are automatically church nursing material.

Often I ruminate concerning the terms nursing and nurse. I recall when I first applied to nursing school and was asked the ultimate questions: why do you want to be a nurse, and what is your definition of nursing? Boldly I answered: "I want to be a nurse because I like helping people, and my definition of nursing was: "helping people when they are in need of assistance." While my answers were not far from the truth, I soon found that nursing incorporates a colossal of tasks; although many of us have performed various nursing tasks unknowingly. Some tasks include: nurturing and caring for a child or love one, teaching one to take their medications appropriately, administering medications, changing diapers, cleaning/dressings wounds, nursing someone ill back to health, and the list goes on and on; still the role play is nursing.

Yes, many of us have taken on nursing roles whether the treatment plan derives from a physician and prescribed medications, the use of over-the-counter-medications (OTC), or simply grandmas' special remedies; the tasks performed are nursing orientated. Often, upon welcoming my nursing students on the first day of class, I generally inform them that *"you are now changing from being a nurse in the home to a more structured form of nursing called professional nursing"*, which in my humble opinion is exactly what professional nursing consist of. Now, let us take a look at the technical or politically correct terminology of the words nurse and nursing.

Defining the Term Nurse?

According to Google.com (2016) the *Noun* meaning of the term nurse is "a person trained to care for the sick or infirm, especially in a hospital. Synonyms: caregiver, Registered Nurse (RN), Licensed Practical Nurse (LPN), nurse practitioner, physician assistant, health care worker" (p.1). The *Verb* meaning of the term nurse is defined as "giving medical and other attention to a sick person. Synonyms: care for, take care of, look after, tend, minister to" (Google.com, 2016, p. 1). Merriam-Webster (2016) defines nurse as "a person who cares for the sick or infirm; *specifically*: a licensed health-care professional who practices independently or is supervised by a physician, surgeon, or dentist and who is skilled in promoting and maintaining health" (p.1).

Defining Professional Nursing?

I attest both professional and church "nursing is an emotionally fulfilling and rewarding career" (Johnson & Johnson, 2016, p.1). Professional nurses: registered nurses (RN's) and license practical nurses (LPN's) perform various roles and according to an organization called The Truth About

Nursing (2002):

Nurses save and improve lives as front line members of the health care delivery team. They independently assess and monitor patients, and taking a holistic approach, determine what patients need to attain and preserve their health. Nurses then provide care and, if needed, alert other health care professionals to assist. For instance, emergency department nurses triage all incoming patients, deciding which are the sickest and in what order they require the attention of other health care professionals. Thus, nurses coordinate care delivery by physicians, nurse practitioners, social workers, physical therapists and others. Nurses assess whether care is successful. If not, they create a different plan of action (p.1).

In general, the American Nurses Association (2016) conceive that "nursing is the protection, promotion, and optimization of health and abilities, prevention of illness and injury, facilitation of healing, alleviation of suffering through the diagnosis and treatment of human response, and advocacy in the care of individuals, families, groups, communities, and populations "(p.1). Many professional nurses work in various churches (known as Parish Nursing), yet this type of nursing is not to be mistaken as the church nurse found in some Baptist

Churches. Let us take a glance at the *Parish Nurse* verses the church nurse participating in some Baptist Churches. In defining any term, because of my love for Christianity, often I seek the Bible for clarity.

Is the Term *Nurse* Mentioned in the Bible?

While the precise term nurse in not mentioned in the Bible, the term deaconess correlates with the meaning of nurse, and is mentioned in the Holy Bible. Merriam-Webster (n.d.) defines the term deaconess as "a woman in some Christian churches who has special duties: a female deacon, or a woman chosen to assist in the church ministry; *specifically*: one in a Protestant order" (p.1). Deaconess comes from "a Greek word *diakonos* (διάκονος), for deacon, meaning a servant or helper and occurs frequently in the Christian New Testament of the Bible. Deaconess traces their roots from the time of Jesus Christ through the 13th century in the West" (Wikipedia, 2016d). The Holy Bible speaks of one individual in particular who was given the title of deaconess.

"Phoebe is named in the New Testament as the first deaconess, and she is noted for opening her home to the sick and needy (Rom. 16:1-2). But Phoebe wasn't the only person to do this. As the church grew, many wealthy widows and matrons established places of comfort for those who were ill" (Laity Services Committee, n.d., p.1). Now let us take a look at the term *nursing* and *church nursing* from a professional and religious perspective.

CHAPTER 2
WHY IS CHURCH NURSING NEEDED?

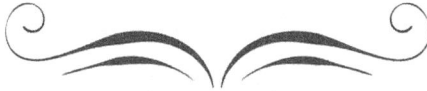

In all organizations auxiliaries and individuals are needed to assist their leader in various roles; lest the leader become burned-out from a tedious/strenuous workload. In addition, the leader is strongest when assistance is rendered. I recall reading in the Bible when one leader chosen by God was informed by his father-in-law that he needed assistance in leading a particular large group of people. I assert that all leaders need assistance with large or small groups in order to lead effectively. In the Holy Bible Moses' Father-in-law (Jethro) instructed him to appoint other individuals to assist him, and it reads:

> And it came to pass on the morrow that Moses sat to judge the people: and the people stood by Moses from the morning unto the evening. And when Moses'

father in law saw all that he did to the people, he said, what is this thing that thou doest to the people? Why sittest thou thyself alone, and all the people stand by thee from morning unto even? And Moses said unto his father in law, because the people come unto me to enquire of God: When they have a matter, they come unto me; and I judge between one and another, and I do make them know the statutes of God, and his laws. And Moses' father in law said unto him, the thing that thou doest is not good. Thou *wilt surely wear away*, both thou, and this people that is with thee: for this thing is *too heavy for thee*; thou art not able to *perform it thyself alone.* Hearken now unto my voice, I will give thee counsel, and God shall be with thee: Be thou for the people to God-ward, that thou mayest bring the causes unto God: And thou shalt teach them ordinances and laws, and shalt shew them the way wherein they must walk, and the work that they must do. Moreover thou shalt provide out of all the people able men, such as fear God, men of truth, hating covetousness; and place such over them, to be rulers of thousands, and rulers of hundreds, rulers of fifties, and rulers of tens: And let them judge the people at all seasons: and it shall be, that every great matter they shall bring unto thee, but every small matter they shall judge: so shall it be easier for thyself, and they shall bear the burden with thee. If thou shalt do this thing, and God command thee so, then thou shalt be able to endure, and all this people shall also go to their place in peace. *So Moses hearkened to the voice of his father in law, and did all that he had said.* And Moses chose able men out of all Israel, and made them heads over the people, rulers of thousands, rulers of hundreds, rulers of fifties, and rulers of tens. And they judged the people at all seasons: the hard cases they brought unto Moses, but every small matter they judged themselves. And Moses let his father in law depart; and he went his way into his own land (Exodus 19: 13-27).

This passage in the Bible confirms when God appoints individuals to perform particular tasks, it is wise for leaders to listen and adhere to God-fearing individuals who are also guided by the Holy Spirit and have their best interest at heart. . . Amen. In essence, the pastors of any church need assistance, and the nurse's guild is just one auxiliary that can assist in this area by caring for those who warrant assistance; rather it's a glass of water to quince their thirst, aid to mend a wound, or whatever the circumstances are, the nurse's guild is an asset in assisting leadership.   In assisting pastors and parishioners, some churches adhere to old standards while other churches have implemented new standards. Now, let us review some duties of a parish nurse.

The Parish Nurse

Many churches throughout the past years use to practice the healing of the whole person (mind, body, and spirit) up until technology progressed narrowing the interest of their parishioners to only the spiritual life, and parting the physical and emotional wellbeing side (Neff, n.d.). Because of the depletion of the whole person wellness in the church, a Lutheran pastor in the 1970's (Dr. Granger Westberg), committed to integrate mind, body and spiritual healing back into the church.   Dr. Westberg's studies and research conducted on the whole person wellness resulted in what is known as the Parish Nurse Ministry (Neff, n.d.). Parish nursing, according to Lueders-Bolwerk (2009):

Also called faith community nurse, is a registered nurse

who serves a church or parish in a *volunteer or paid position*. Most often, parish nurses are connected to a congregation, serving in a variety of ways, promoting health for the whole person. Parish nurses act as health educators, personal health counselors, health advocates, referral agents, coordinators of volunteers and integrators of faith and wellness . . . in addition to, practice nursing on an independent level under the standards of faith community nursing and licensure in our states. In health care today . . . the parish nurses are sensitive to how . . . patients are affected on a holistic level. For example, nurses understand that breast cancer not only affects a woman on a physical level, but it significantly affects her spirit, mind and interpersonal relationships. The parish nurse in meeting the health care needs of all people . . . use the church as a base for health care. Parish nurses assist members in their physical, emotional and spiritual wellbeing. A study . . . conducted on 82 parish nurses revealed various activities parish nurses participate in. For instance, 80 percent of parish nurses screen for hypertension on "*Blood Pressure Sundays.*" Others present educational workshops on health topics such as breast cancer, diabetes, bone health, depression, advance directives and the like. Fifty percent of those surveyed coordinated health fairs, bridging resources from the community to church members. Many parish nurses have hosted flu shot clinics and blood drives on church sites, while others have facilitated support groups for grief and weight loss, counsel congregational members on medications, lifestyles, diagnostic tests to improve health and well-being. Visits to the homebound and members living in nursing homes comprise about 60 percent of parish nurses' activities (p. 30-31).

As one can see parish nursing is different from church nursing in relationship to the nurse's guild as orchestrated in some Baptist Churches.

Church Nursing Definition and Establishment

Church nursing is a volunteered service by parishioners of an organization to assist their pastor, associate clergy staff, and parishioners during various services held in their establishment or a visiting church. Church nursing commonly exists in African American churches (mainly Baptist) and have been in existence for over 70 years. The nurses' guild regularly works congruently with the usher board in tending to the needs of the parishioners (Evers, 2012) and visitors. The nurses' guild staff, in addition to tending to the needs of the clergy, members, and visitors, may render minor first-aid services' to anyone in the congregation when needed. In the past, churches only had a few nurses to perform these roles; however, churches upon gaining more nurses formed what we know today as the nurses' guild and in some churches the nurse's guild now include more non-emergency responsibilities (Evers, 2012).

General Qualifications of a Church Nurse

From a personal perspective, the church nurse' first priority is to love and serve God. In addition, the church nurse must have a loving spirit to care for others from the heart, willing to care for the pastor, other clergy, and all saints in the church "distributing to the necessity of saints; given to hospitality" (Romans 12:13). According to Greater Progressive Baptist Church (2012), nurses on the guild are to help address the basic physical needs of the church and the community. Their vision is to provide care, compassion, and comfort to others. Individuals considering church nursing should have experience or interests in the health care field, and have a passion for serving. The church nurse spiritual gifts includes:

skills, traits, ability to show compassion, effectively interact with diverse groups of all ages, and maintains confidentiality of all in which they encounter (Greater Progressive Baptist Church, 2012). Although some churches allow members to *just have a desire* to be a church nurse others prefer their nurses' guild members to have acquired some type of credentials in the medical field. For the most part, the church nurse qualifications include a desire and willingness to render services to the pastor and parishioners. Many churches call church nursing a ministry or a nurse's guild.

Typically, their role or mission is to minister (*verb meaning: provide or give help*) to the pastor (before and after preaching), tend to other ministers on the rostrum. The assigned nurse(s) for a given Sunday should accompany the pastor or assigned minister to all services, while tending to their needs as in serving water, beverages, providing a handkerchief, towel, robe, mints, or whatever the pastor requests. While some pastors and ministers prefer to change into a cape after preaching, others prefer changing their shirts (often they will bring these items with them). Services include Sunday mornings, Sunday afternoon services, funerals, special events, and services conducted throughout the week. In regards to additional church nurses' duties: nurses are to perform duties assigned by the pastor, provide first aid to the ill or injured, when needed provide support to ushers during church services (especially in assisting emotionally-aroused individuals), and maintaining the upkeep of the nursing office/health room. Nurses on the guild and ushers *should always control crowds* when someone has fainted, appear unresponsive, or when attending to an individual who becomes ill in the congregation. Only the older professional nurses on the guild should attend to parishioners appearing unresponsive. Younger nurses (while very useful) may not have had training in this area.

CHAPTER 3
WHAT AGE IS FEASIBLE FOR CHURCH NURSING?

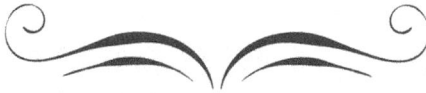

Many churches train youth (wearing candy stripes uniforms) to work on the nurse's guild, while other churches solicit teenagers and adults. On a personal level, I strongly believe in training children to render service for the Lord at a very young age for any auxiliary. My philosophy comes from the Word of God which states to "Train up a child in the way he should go: and when he is old, he will not depart from it" (Proverbs 22:6). Who knows, perhaps they may follow this path and become a professional nurse. In addition, I strongly believe that the age in which a child is able to reason, understands logic, confesses that Jesus is Lord, and is accepted as a member of the chosen church is the appropriate age to allow them to join the nurses' guild if they so desire. As a past president of a nurses' guild, youth were allowed to join at an early age, and they were very attentive and great in performing their duties. I really enjoyed working with them and highly appreciated their service. Below is a past picture of the nurses' guild in which I was blessed to lead; since then they are all grown-up and have families of their own.

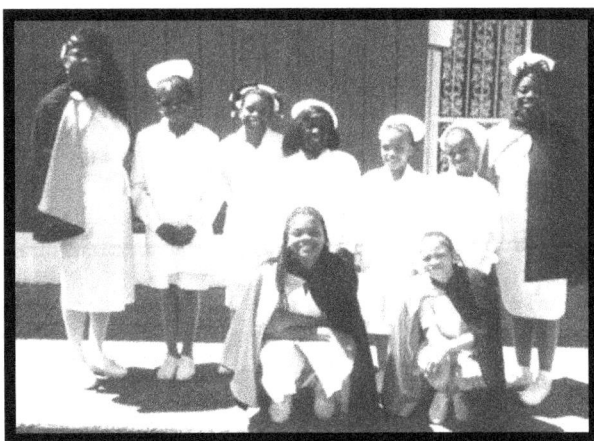

Ultimately, the age for individuals desiring to be on the Nurse's Guild is established by the residing Pastor of the church. All things must be done "decently and in order" (1st Corinthians 14:40), therefore the pastor will spearhead the Nurse's Guild auxiliary; setting the standards and qualifications. Sometimes the Pastor will appoint a president over the Nurse's Guild and instruct this individual to implement standards and may then change or revise them. While age is at the discretion of the residing pastor of the assembly so is the determination of the gender of the nursing guild.

Can Men Join The Nurses' Guild?

Over the past years, church nursing have been adopted for adult females yet, some churches now allow both genders to join the guild. Again, in any organization whether it be businesses or churches, one must abide by the rules and regulations set forth by the overseers, pastors, or administration. In my humble opinion, men should be allowed to join nurse' guild, but as previously stated the decision is determined by the pastor of the church. Surprising to many, 2000 years ago *men were the first nurses*, and *nursing schools were for men only.* Historically speaking, only men were considered clean enough to become nurses, and the world's first nursing school for men was established 250 B.C. in India (Thunderwolf, 2006).

While men were dominating nursing schools, Florence Nightingale (known as the founder of modern nursing; the lady with the lamp) in 1860 established her own school of nursing (at St. Thomas's Hospital) in London (Wikipedia, 2016b). Of course, Florence Nightingale school of Nursing was for women only. In remembrance of Nightingale and her contributions to the nursing profession, nursing schools nationwide (LPN's and

RN's) continue to honor her by allowing their newly graduating nurses (in pinning ceremonies) to recite the Nightingale Pledge. This pledge is a statement of ethics and principles of the nursing profession; yet some of the pledge can be employed for church nursing. One can review the Florence Nightingale Pledge at the end of Chapter Seven (7). Although Nightingale opened the door for women to enroll in nursing schools, men dominated the nursing field establishing nursing schools as early as the 1800's.

In fact, two in particular were established in New York (Mills Nursing School and St. Vincent's Hospital School for men) in 1888. Furthermore, women did not become the chosen gender for the nursing profession until 1901, in which the Army Nurse Corps was formed allowing only women to serve as nurses. Still in 1914 the Pennsylvania Hospital opened separate schools of nursing (one for women and one for men) to attend (Thunderwolf, 2006). Currently there is an increase in the enrollment of men in nursing schools due to a predicted nursing shortage in the upcoming years, changes in a U.S. Supreme Court case in 1981 deeming *no allowance of men enrollment into nursing school unconstitutional*, the expansion of nursing rolls and elevated pay (especially nurse practitioners and nurse anesthetists (approximately $162,900 annually), and job stability found in the nursing profession (U.S. Census Bureau, 2013).

Still the nursing profession is growing and rewarding, "there were 3.5 million employed nurses in 2011, about 3.2 million whom were females and 330, 000 males" (U.S. Census Bureau, 2013, p.2). Men are not only enrolling in professional nursing school, but are joining the nurses' guild in some churches. Again, it is the solemn authority of the residing pastor to set the gender status for the nurses' guild in their organization as with standards for the guild. While, standards, policies, procedures, and qualifications vary from one organization to another, some general qualifications are listed for all projected and current nurses' on a nurses' guild.

Old and New Standards for the Church Nurse

In addition to assisting the clergy and their needs, some areas of assisting parishioners (in the past) included tending to members who became ill or has fainted. In agreement with Evers (2012), I recall seeing nurses run to members who had fainted with what we called (back in the day) smelling sauce (in actuality, it is known as smelling salt. Smelling salts, "also known as ammonia inhalants, spirit of hartshorn, or sal volatile are chemical compounds used for arousing consciousness"

(Wikipedia, 2016a) and continues to be used today in health, household, and baby care; nevertheless, *are not used* in many churches. Smelling salts (ammonium carbonate) have been employed since Roman times and are also used as stimulants in athletic competitions to arouse athletes for better performance; yet, they *have been banned* in nearly all boxing competitions (Wikipedia, 2016a).

While no side effects have been reported from the use of smelling salts (generally small amounts), high ammonia gas administered in large concentrations for prolonged periods can become fatal and the use of high concentrated ammonia inhalants may burn the nasal cavity and oral mucosa (Wikipedia, 2016a). Most importantly," the use of ammonia smelling salts to revive people injured during sport, is not recommended because it may inhibit or delay a proper and through neurological assessment by a healthcare professional" (Wikipedia, 2016a, p. 1). In my humble opinion, as a church nurse and professional Registered Nurse (RN), I highly protest against the use of smelling salts in church nursing.

The current standards for the layperson employed in church nursing in regards to someone fainting is to simply give the person air (do not crowd the individual), fan them, call out their name, and ask if they are alright. When there is a professional medical person around, let them assess the individual and follow their directives. If the individual does not respond, call 911 immediately and let the professional or other trained staff in CPR start the process immediately. While some individuals may faint and are revived, others may not. Try to remove the person away from the crowd immediately and as quietly as possible (The National Baptist Convention, 2014). Listed below is pertinent information regarding fainting. According to Jaret (2017):

Many people feel lightheaded every once in a while, so lightheaded that they may faint -- that is, pass out momentarily. Fainting is not the same as being asleep or unconscious. When a person faints, it's usually temporary and the person can be revived in a few minutes . . . Fainting often results when blood flow to the brain is temporarily inadequate. This can happen as a result of stress, grief, overheating, dehydration, exhaustion, or illness; fainting may also occur after taking certain medications. Standing for an extended period in very hot weather -- especially with locked knees -- can also make people pass out. Inactivity can cause blood to settle in the lower parts of the body, reducing the amount of blood flowing into the brain . . . Soldiers standing at attention for long periods are prone to fainting, . . . Certain medications can lower blood pressure to a level that will trigger fainting. People with diabetes can sometimes lose consciousness if their blood sugar levels are too high or too low. Many people recover very quickly from a brief loss of consciousness without any harmful consequences. However, on some occasions, fainting can signal a medical emergency. Don't treat fainting as minor unless you're certain there is no serious underlying cause . . . You may be able to tell when someone is about to faint. The warning signs include: pale, cool, and sweaty skin, lightheadedness or dizziness, a slow pulse, nausea, frequent yawning, feeling of restlessness, tightness in the chest, and palpitations (p.1).

In the event of an emergency, such as one becoming unconscious and there is a professional individual on the nurses' guild (someone trained in CPR) or someone in the congregation, allow that individual to assess and care for the parishioner. If none are trained in CPR, call 911 immediately. So often people assume because one is wearing *white* they are trained in medical emergencies. While having all individuals on the nurse' guild trained in CPR is idea, it is not mandated in most Baptist churches. For the most part, nurses wear *white* in remembrance of the historical nursing uniform being white and the meaning of the *color white.* *Still, church* nursing and professional nursing is about God, not about exploiting a white uniform. My philosophy: *a uniform does not make the nurse, the nurse makes the uniform.*

CHAPTER 4
DRESS CODE FOR THE CHURCH NURSE

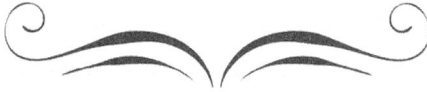

So what about this white uniform? All over the world nurses' professionally (even students in most nursing schools) have changed from the color of white to various colors representing nursing. So why not church nursing? Good question; many nursing schools have changed their color from white to various colors at the request of their nursing students and site representatives.   Many professional nurses' colors changed from white to other colors because of the nurses preferences in not wanting to wear white (stating it gets dirty too quickly) and because of professional color codes resulting in identity of staff members working in the health field.

However, one has yet to see the various colors representing the nurses' guilds in the Baptist churches; currently, they are still wearing white. Personally, I love the portrayal of white representing nurses; in my honest opinion white symbolizes significance. According to the Bible Study Site (n.d.), the color white is the presence of all the light in the visible spectrum. When it enters our eyes, it stimulates all of our cone cells that God made light sensitive. Snow and clouds appear like it because almost all of the light from the sun is reflected by water (either frozen or liquid), with only a small amount of the visible spectrum absorbed. This color, in the Bible and in today's society, is typically associated with purity, things that are good, innocence, honesty, and cleanliness.

The Meaning of the Color White in the Bible

In the King James Version (KJV) Bible, the word 'white' occurs seventy-five times, twenty-nine of which are in the New Testament. It is the most frequently mentioned color in not only the entire word of God but also the New Testament. It is the third most referenced color in the Old Testament, behind blue (50) and red (47). The color white's used in Scripture lends itself to symbolically meaning righteousness (Daniel 7:9, Matthew 17:2, Mark 9:3, Luke 9:29, Revelation 1:12 - 14, 6:11, 19:8, 20:11) or pretending to be so (Revelation 6:2), or made pure (Daniel 11:35, 12:10, Psalm 51:7, Isaiah 1:18, Revelation 3:18, 7:9, 13 - 14), it also symbolizes wisdom (Revelation 1:14), holiness or dedication to God (2Chronicles 5:12, Mark 16:5, John 20:12, Acts 1:10, Revelation 4:4, 19:14) or joy (Ecclesiastes 9:8) . . . (The Bible Study Site, n.d.).

I recall the Word of God speaking about my Savior Jesus Christ (prophecy) riding on a *white horse* as mentioned in Revelations. Everything about my Lord and Savior is Good. This book converses about two prophetic horses, one of the horses representing God and it states: "And I saw heaven opened, and behold a white horse; and he that sat upon him was called Faithful and True, and in righteousness he doth judge and make war. His eyes were as a flame of fire, and on his head were many crowns; and he had a name written, that no man knew, but he himself. And he was clothed with vesture dipped in blood: and his name is called The Word of God" (Revelation 19:11-13).

Webster's Dictionary (1913) defines the word white as, having the color of purity, free from spot or blemish, or from guilt or pollutions; innocent, pure. According to surveys in Europe and the United States, white is the color most often associated with perfection, the good, honesty, cleanliness, the beginning, the new, neutrality, and exactitude. White is an important color for almost all world religions (Wikipedia, 2017). Yes, the nursing uniform has changed dramatically. Yet it is a known fact that nurses did not start out wearing white uniforms.

The First Nursing Uniform Wasn't White

In fact, according to Wikipedia (2016d):

The first nurse uniforms were derived from the nun's habit. Before the 19th century, nuns took care of sick and injured people so it was obvious that trained lay nurses might copy the nun's habit as they have adopted ranks like "Sister." One of Florence Nightingale's first students (Miss van Rensselaer) designed the original uniform for the students at Miss Nightingale's school of nursing. Before the 1940s minor changes occurred in the uniform. The clothing consisted of a mainly blue outfit. Hospitals were free to determine the style of the nurse uniform, including the nurse's cap which exists in many variants . . . In Britain, the national uniform (or simply "national") was designed with the advent of the National Health Service (NHS) in 1948, and the Newcastle dress. From the 1960s open necks began to appear. In the 1970s, white disposable paper caps replaced cotton ones; in the 1980s, plastic aprons displaced the traditional ones and outerwear began to disappear. From the 1990s, *scrubs* became popular in Britain, having first appeared in the USA; however, some nurses in Britain continue to wear dresses, although some NHS trusts have removed them in favor of scrubs as in many other countries (p.1).

The White Uniform

For the most part, the color white is still employed in numerous Baptist churches in relationship to the nurse's guild. Female nurses in many churches still wear the traditional white dress uniforms (emulating the once dominated white uniform worn by professional nurses) and sometimes white lab jackets or lab coats, while some females on the nurses' guild have resulted to wearing white scrub tops and pants with the lab jackets. Basically, it is a matter of each organization's preference. Some nurses on the nurses' guild have added the navy blue capes, which exemplifies an even more professional look for the nurses' guild. Often the capes are worn for special occasions (although some nurses wear them all the time) as in: visiting other churches, the Pastor's anniversary, and funerals.

Generally the cape is folded back on one side except for funerals; in which it is closed. The male uniform generally consists of white scrub tops, pants, and a lab jacket or long lab coat. Lab jackets or lab coats may be worn by either gender. The long lab coats are often worn in the winter since they hold heat. Yes, the white uniforms portray a very professional appearance especially when they are clean. Nurse's uniforms should be clean at all times especially in the house of God.

How to Care for the White Uniform

For the most part, white uniforms over time tend to turn dingy in color; why is this? Many uniforms are made up of various materials and must be cleaned only by the specific instructions provided on the label. Listed below are some pointers in keeping your uniform looking brand new and bright:

- Follow specific cleaning instructions for your particular uniform material.
- Always separate the colors from the whites.
- Add baking soda to your wash to bring back the whiteness.
- Do not add bleach to your white uniform.
- Never overload your washer when washing whites.

- Use plenty of cold water to wash away the detergent.
- It is better to let your white uniform air dry/ put on hanger.
- If in a hurry for drying set the dryer on permanent press or cool.

So much for keeping the uniform clean, now let us dab into the significance of wearing dark undergarments.

Under Garments Pertaining to the Nurses' Guild

Women and men church nurses' undergarments should be of dark colors (black or navy); as the lining of undergarments are not seen when worn under white clothing. If a female is wearing dark underwear (black or navy), she can wear a white slip; as the dark underwear will not show through the white slip. The wearing of *thongs* are not appropriate or necessary; however, stockings are. Women should always wear white stockings or pantyhose with their nursing uniform; never bear legs.

Stockings and Socks

Women' stockings or pantyhose should always be white and without holes, blemish, or ruins. The prudent church nurse always keeps an extra pair of white stockings on hand or buys the white nursing support hose which sometimes last for years; these pantyhose not only serve the purpose of being in uniform but also support your legs professionally. They are available online at many stores and in uniform stores nationwide. Of course they cost a little more than the usual white pantyhose but because of their support and viability they are worth it.

Being a church nurse (and in the nursing profession) for years, one can attest that one pair of any nursing support pantyhose will last at least two years; at least mine did and they give extra support to the lower extremities while standing for long periods of time. Support hose are cheaper online; generally ranging in price from $9-$12 dollars. They are also available in knee- highs and thigh- highs; depending on the length in which one desires to accommodate their nursing uniform. For women on nurse's guilds who wear pants, the knee-high white stockings are most appropriate. Men on the other hand, are to wear white socks or support white socks for men. In addition to good support hose or socks, one should always wear comfortable nursing shoes.

Shoes for the Nurses' Guild

Women should wear white nursing shoes that are comfortable in the event they have to stand for long periods of time. Nursing shoes should always be clean and without holes or a worn-out look. Most nursing shoes can be wiped clean with just soap and water (many are made of plastic for the summer months), or one can use white shoe polish. If the nursing shoe has shoestrings, they should also be washed or polished. While some nursing shoes are very expensive, many are now inexpensive, comfortable, and available at many stores. In fact, I have purchased several pairs for under $10. Tip: Some shoes while are not called nursing shoes, are very appropriate to wear (not gym shoes) with the nursing uniform. *High heel white shoes are not appropriate* and should not be worn with the white nursing uniform, neither are they comfortable. Working on the nurses' guild is a Godly duty to serve, not a fashion show. Repeat: In my Father's House, "Let all things be done decently and in order" (1st Corinthians 14:40). Mens' white nursing shoes are available nationwide or they can purchase some white loafers which equally appropriate while dressed in the nurses' uniform. In covering the appropriate uniform attire for members on the nurses' guild, the uniform will not be complete without the embellishment of jewelry.

Jewelry While in Uniform

For many years, the jewelry protocol for nursing schools and church nursing was small post earrings, a wedding ring, and a wrist watch while in uniform. Still in most nursing schools students are allowed to only wear one (1) post pair of earrings, a wedding ring, and wrist watch with the rationales that jewelry around the neck has the potential of falling into a patient's mouth, the patient may grab it, and the notion that jewelry are considered fomites (objects that are likely to carry infections; Farlex, 2017). Nursing overall (professional and church nursing) continues to change, and as time passes various trends have evolved with the church nurses' regalia. Some church nurses, instead of wearing post earrings now wear a mixture of jewelry as in matching white sets (earrings, necklace, and bracelets) of various lengths and styles.

While the jewelry sets dress up the uniform (on a personal note) it appears gaudy and takes away from the sincerity of the nurses' guild. Nonetheless, one must remember, this is church nursing (not professional nursing) and many love to dress up on Sundays. Still, some guilds implement specific standards regarding jewelry while in uniform such as post or button earrings (without the necklace or bracelet). When in doubt, follow the protocols of your church or organization. Now let us review the nursing cap.

Nursing Caps for the Nurses' Guild

One could question why do I need to wear a nursing cap while serving on the nurses' guild, even the professional nurses do not wear them? Answer, the nursing cap is part of the nursing uniform for women; and has been worn by female professional nurses (emulated by nursing guilds) for many years. In fact, according to Early (2016):

> The nurse's cap originated in the early Christian Era, as a head covering for deaconesses that cared for the sick. During the 1800's, head coverings evolved into the more familiar white cap that was first used by Florence Nightingale. Around 1874, the Bellevue Training School in New York City adopted a special nursing cap to identify nurses who had graduated from Bellevue. Other nursing schools also developed unique caps as a way to identify the graduate nurse and her school of

nursing (p. 1).

In essence, the nursing cap mimics the nursing profession even though professional nurses no longer wear them. Yet, the nursing cap (in my humble opinion) is one part of the uniform that church nurses appear proud to wear. The nursing cap, just as the white uniform should be clean at all times. Some nurses wash their caps in the washing machine on the gentle cycle; while others wash them by hand. On a personal note, the cap can also be cleaned with shoe polish. Hint: keeping the cap in a nursing cap bag (inexpensive online; around $6) keeps them from turning dull in color. Nursing caps are available in various styles with variable price ranges. One should always comply with their church as to what style they are to purchase. Some churches have resulted to seamstress making personalized nursing caps embroidered with their church name or acronyms representing their church. In addition to the cap being worn with pride, so are personalized nursing badges.

Badges for the Nurses' Guild

Name tags/badges come in various colors, shapes, and sizes. Badges for the nurses' guild often displays the church name, the nurse' name, the auxiliary name, and sometimes the pastor's name. Some pastors may have the nurses' on the guild who possess health care credentials or certifications put their initials aside their name on their badge. Name badges can be expensive when ordering from stores that charge per letter. Ordering online, one can search for cheaper badges of good quality that does not charge per letter. Salient point for female nurses: keep your badge in your nursing cap bag (if you possess one) to avoid leaving it at home, or keep them in the nursing office at your church (providing the church has a nursing office). One should value their church badge as if it is their badge used at their employment. Praise God, we are now in full uniform, now let us access other issues encountered by nurses on the guild such as over the counter (OTC) medications.

CHAPTER 5
THE NURSES' GUILD AND (ON-SITE) OTC MEDICATIONS

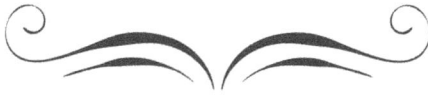

Many churches allow their nurses on the guild to give parishioners over the counter (OTC) meds such as aspirin, Tums, and many others. This practice has always been a great concern of mine. Although, some health care facilities allow non-nursing personnel to pass meds (as in some assisted living centers) I am sure they have policies, procedures, protocols, and some type of law abiding standards that allow them to practice in the manner. Nevertheless, I contend that only professional nurses should administer medications (OTC and prescribed) under the guidance of a physician. There are exceptions to this rule for some *advanced practice nurses* who have the qualifications and the authority to write certain prescriptions which varies from state to state (Nurses Service

Organization, 2017).

Professional nurses can however, take verbal orders (while working in a healthcare facility) from a physician via phone in an emergency situation, but even this verbal order must be written in a specific timeframe. When professional nurses administer medications to any individual without a physician's order (OTC and prescribed meds), they are stepping out of their scope of practice and clinical privileges (Nurses Service Organization, 2017). In doing so one stands the risks of jeopardizing the parishioner, your church, and yourself in the capacity of continuing to practice nursing; in addition to potential malpractice lawsuits which may lead to criminal charges (remember, you are not a physician practicing medicine). The prudent professional nurse ascertains their *liability insurance is in good standing* no matter where they practice. We are living in a society in which people are desensitized to almost everything and we must expect the unexpected. We as Christians in loving our church family must remain obedient to The Word which reads, "Behold, I send you forth as sheep in the midst of wolves: be ye therefore wise as serpents, and harmless as doves" (Matthew 10:16).

All professional nurses (on the nursing guild at

churches or working in health care facilities) must adhere to standards under your state and federal laws, and your Nurse Practice Act (Nurses Service Organization, 2017). While it is not uncommon that many professional nurses (working on a nurses' guild or in general) have given OTC medications to their friends or family members and have not faced a lawsuit because something contraindicating happened, *is it worth the risk?* Often one gives their friends and family members OTC medications and even some prescribed medications without doing a thorough assessment . . . as in asking *if they are allergic to certain foods or medications. Be careful!*

Professional nurses on the nurses' guilds (after contacting a physician and given a verbal order to proceed with medications) must remember the five (5) rights when administering medications taught in nursing school: 1. The right drug, 2. The right patient, 3. The right dose, 4. The right route, and 5. The right time. In addition, the professional nurse must always stay within their scope of practice, no matter what they do (Nurses Service Organization, 2017). Often parishioners ask me for OTC medications and I simply inform them that I cannot administer any meds to them because of my professional license and standards. However, many churches are adamant about keeping OTC Medications on hand and allow the parishioners to self-service themselves.

It's not uncommon that when OTC medications *are not available* in the nurses' office the parishioners frequently ask other parishioners for OTC medications; while I inform others of the same rules concerning giving others OTC medications, some churches continue to give out OTC medications. When this happens, I tend to assess the medication cabinet to assure that there are *not expired* medications on board (in some cases, many are) and if they are expired I will throw them out. Nonetheless, there are exceptions to this rule for professional nurses in giving medications in the event of an emergency.

Professional Nurses on the Guild *Can Give* Meds in Emergencies

Professional nurses on the guild may administer medications to parishioners in the event of an emergency and if the parishioner has their medication available. According to Nurses Service Organization (2017):

If you provide emergency care to a patient outside of your place of employment, however, a different standard applies. According to Joanne Sheehan, JD, RN, BSN, an attorney with Friedman, Newman, Levy, Sheehan and Carolan in Fairfield, CT, every state has Good Samaritan laws that protect healthcare providers from liability if they provide emergency care in good faith. Such care would include giving a man who had a heart attack nitroglycerin if he had it with him, for example. These laws have certain "gray" areas and vary slightly from state to state. So it is up to you to familiarize yourself with and understand those laws in your state (p.1).

While administering OTC medications are not idea or prudent of the church nurse, there are other functions in which nurses' on the guild can assist their clergy members and parishioners with minimal instructions, by acquiring minor certifications, and learning to use certain equipment. Pertinent equipment is needed for all nurses on the guild to assess parishioners and individuals in the event of emergency and non-emergency situations effectively.

CHAPTER 6
PERTINENT EQUIPMENT NEEDED ON SITE

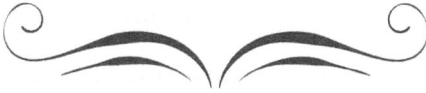

In all cases, for any nurse to assist others effectively it is imperative that nurses' have access to viable pertinent equipment. If at all possible, a room should be provided for the nurses alone. The first item of importance is a sink with good running cold and hot water (to wash hands and dishes). The sink should be large enough to accommodate a dish rack to dry dishes. A refrigerator is another item needed to keep beverages cold and to house ice. Another item of importance is a microwave to assist in warming beverages and other items if needed. Churches providing a storage cabinet large enough to store drinking glasses, water pitchers, Kleenex, paper towels, a nurses' log/referral book, and other equipment will highly accommodate and assist the church nurse. Other tools that may benefit church nurses are: a first aid-kit, blood pressure apparatus (wrist or arm) adjustable to fit all sizes, glucometer, pulse oximeter, thermometer, hot/cold packs, a walker, a wheelchair, cane, and if possible an automatic external defibrillator (AED).

Beneficial Tools for the Nursing Office

The most powerful and beneficial tool nurses on the guild can display is the protection of all from the transmission of germs and bacteria by always washing their hands before and after tasks.   Hand washing is the number one defense against the spread of disease and should always be performed. If no sink with running water and soap is available one should have a bottle of hand sanitizer available at all times (especially when visiting other churches).   Other powerful tools that are beneficial for church nurses are the continuity in reading and gaining knowledge from the Word of God (strengthens the mind, body, and soul) and researching and retaining knowledge related to first-aid that will assist self and others in the event of emergency and non-emergency matters.

Enhancing Ones' Knowledge as a Beneficial Tool

We should always study the Word of God which is a lamp unto our feet, and a light unto our path (Psalm 119: 105;

paraphrased). God wants His stewards to be knowledgeable concerning all things (I Thessalonians 4:13), this includes learning about His Word and services we are rendering in His Name (on the job and in church). As taught in professional nursing school; the fear of the unknown increase anxiety (Savva, 2017). In essence, when one is not trained or uncertain what to do in an event of an emergency or non-emergency they may become anxious. When in doubt, seek assistance. While some individuals are unable to attend college, with the World Wide Web (WWW) and Google access there is diminutive excuses for *not knowing*, in particular concerning basic first-aid and CPR. In addition, You-Tube has trustworthy learning tools to assist one in learning to efficiently operate apparatuses such as blood pressure machines, thermometers, glucometers, pulse oximeters, and practically anything else.

Reading is fundamental, and nurses on the guild possessing some knowledge concerning first-aid is highly favorable. Being in the medical field for a period of time has allowed me to encounter many individuals (in my humble opinion), who should have gone to medical, law, or nursing school due to their large knowledge base. These individuals (while not interested in going to college) obtained their knowledge from reading books, magazines, and researching data from scholarly and reliable internet sites.

While the professional nurse is expected to have a large knowledge base, I contend when one encounters one wearing an all-white uniform (in church nursing or professional nursing) they believe the individual possesses a good knowledge base. Why not gain knowledge concerning skills that will enhance your tasks on any auxiliary, especially in the service of the Lord? Surely, one is eager to gain degrees and certifications to enhance their skills serving in the secular world, why not improve one's skills to enhance serving in the House of God? Why not study the Word of God more to strengthen our faith and knowledge base, in an effort to strengthen our brethren (Luke: 22:32). As Christians we are to study to show ourselves "approved unto God, a workman that needeth not to be ashamed, rightly dividing the word of truth" (2nd Timothy 2:15); this is not only in the Word of God, but in all things. In meeting the needs of parishioners, offering valid information (even if it's a referral) is very much accommodating. Church nurses in meeting the needs of parishioners can provide health informational pamphlets concerning various manners and apparatus which will highly assist them in non-emergency and emergency needs. The nurse on the guild, above all things must service parishioners and other with the right attitude.

The Right Attitude as a Beneficial Tool

As a Christian church nurse we must love everyone and treat them with respect, dignity, kindness, and a humble attitude. Yes, attitude is important. The author Charles Swindoll quoted that attitude will "make or break a company . . . a church . . . a home. Swindoll goes on to say that, "I am convinced that life is 10% what happens to me and 90% how I react to it. While it is certain that people may provoke one to anger, we are to "be angry and sin not" (Ephesians 4:26) and continue to love, care, and forgive others. In spite of individuals inappropriate attitudes we must be obedience to the Word of God; "Therefore all things whatsoever ye would that men should do to you, do ye even so to them: for this is the law and the prophets" (Matthew 7:12). Remaining humble in spirit is of God and Christian like. We must be "wise as serpents, and harmless as doves" (Matthew 10:16) in all services rendered. Other tools that may be of value to assist the church nurse are listed below.

The Nursing Office and Apparatuses

Nursing Office

In the event an extra room is available in the church, it should be employed as a nursing's quarters or office. Included in this room should be a roll-a-way or twin bed which is necessary for individuals who may need to lie down in privacy. In this instance, the professional nurse or certified medical personnel (on the nurse's guild; if available) can conduct a full assessment (in privacy) in an effort of not breaching the health insurance probability and accountability act of 1996 (HIPPA) laws regarding confidentiality. In the event of a true emergency call 911. If the parishioner has sustained any minor injuries the first aid kit may be of value to the assessor.

First-Aid Kit

Nurses' guilds in purchasing a *First Aid Kit* allow the nurse to readily assess minor or common injuries generally acquired in the organization. Nurses on the guild who are trained in first-aid (generally offered with the CPR Training) are aware of the contents found in these kits. A basic first aid kit may include: antibiotic ointment, antiseptic towelettes, adhesive plastic bandages (Band-Aids; different sizes), wound closures, disposable cold/hot packs, disposable gloves, sterile gauze pads, non-sterile bandage, medical tape, first aid guide, and an accident report form. First aid kits are variable in prices and contents; generally the higher the cost of the kit the more contents enclosed. Always check the expiration dates of the materials enclosed before using. Some first aid kits include first aid manual-flyers to display in the nursing office/quarters which recap on some first aid skills concerning minor injuries. Flyers displaying other significant instructions as in taking blood pressures are also helpful.

Blood Pressure Apparatus

It is not uncommon for parishioners to ask a nurse on the guild to take their blood pressure. While taking blood pressures can be easily taught to others (using a wrist device) it is highly recommended that individuals trained regarding the pathophysiology; means whereby such condition develops and progresses (or the significance of the meaning of blood pressure) should take them. Often parishioners may experience problems with their blood pressure which is expressed in measurements of two numbers. The top number (systolic; range 90-120) measures the pressure in your arteries during the contraction of your heart muscle, while the bottom number (diastolic; range 60-80) measures the pressure when your heart muscle is between beats. The normal blood pressure is 120/80 and when this number is higher than the normal range, it indicates that the heart is overworking to pump blood to the rest of the body (American Heart Association, 2017). Some individuals may need reassurance in knowing if their blood pressure is high or low, and may ask a nurse on the guild to take their pressure. Preferably, blood pressures should be taken by individuals trained to take them; make sure the blood pressure apparatus is working effectively.

A blood pressure apparatus (wrist or arm) adjustable to fit all sizes is always feasible for the nurses' quarters in reassuring parishioners that their blood pressure is within the normal range. Some parishioners are not fortunate to have their own blood pressure apparatus in their homes and may ask the nurse to take their blood pressure. Still, a professional nurse or medical personnel (on the guild) should ascertain the blood pressure apparatus is properly working and that the right size cuff is applied (inappropriate cuff sizes will give an inaccurate readings).

When in doubt (as to if the blood pressure apparatus is working properly) always check both arms (if applicable; some individuals can only have their blood pressure taken in one arm due to medical devices inserted or medical disorders). Generally, the blood pressure reading in one arm is not too much different in the other, unless there is underlying medical disorder with the individual. Assess if the individual has a history of hypertension/hypotension, and inquire if the individual takes prescribed medications for these disorders. If the individuals' blood pressure reading is not within the normal range (120/80; some contend 110/70) refer the individual to their primary care physician or the emergency room. The professional nurse should always document abnormal findings and referrals (follow-up recommendations) given to the parishioner in a log book that is kept under lock and key for at least 3 years for references. Another device that may be useful for nurses' on the guild and accessible in the office is the glucometer.

Glucometer

All individuals trained in using the glucometer (in addition to washing their hands prior) must use disposable gloves.   The glucometer involves needle puncture and gloves are used to decrease the risk of spreading bacteria, disease, and germs. The use of non-latex gloves is idea in implementing all procedures requiring gloves for protection, and the prevention of allergic reactions on behalf of individuals known to have latex allergies (or individuals unaware if they are allergic to latex). Individuals known to have allergic reactions to latex should avoid contact (if at all possible) with latex products, which may cause severe to critical outcomes (American College of Allergy, Asthma, & Immunology, 2014; Soares, 2015).

Dangers of Latex Allergies

Individuals experiencing latex allergic reactions may have "asthma symptoms of wheezing, chest tightness and difficulty breathing. Symptoms begin within minutes after exposure to products containing latex. The most severe latex allergy can result in anaphylaxis, a serious allergic reaction involving severe breathing difficulty and/or fall in blood pressure; shock" (Ansell, 2017, p.1). If only latex gloves are available, always ask the individual before pulling out the gloves (to take their blood glucose level) if they are allergic to latex.

The glucometer is valid in measuring blood sugar levels when a person may be experiencing low/high blood sugars levels. The normal blood sugar range is 80-130 (American Diabetes Association, 2017a). Low blood sugar levels are 70mg/dl (milligram/deciliter) and below.

Signs and symptoms of low blood sugars (hypoglycemia) vary with each individual and may appear quickly (American Diabetes Association, 2017b) such as:

Signs and Symptoms of Low (Glucose Levels) Blood Sugars	
Shakiness	Nervousness/anxiety
Sweating	Chills and clamminess
Irritability/impatience	Confusion (including delirium)
Rapid/fast heartbeat	Lightheadedness/ dizziness
Hunger and nausea	Sleepiness
Blurred/impaired vision	Tingling or numbness in the lips or tongue

Headaches	Weakness or fatigue
Anger	Stubbornness or sadness
Lack of coordination	Nightmares or crying out during sleep
Seizures and unconsciousness	
(American Diabetes Association, 2017b, p. 1).	

High blood sugars levels are known as hyperglycemia. "Hyperglycemia happens when the body has too little insulin or when the body can't use insulin properly" (American Diabetes Association, 2017c, p.1). Some signs and symptoms of hyperglycemia (also variable in individuals) are: high blood glucose, high levels of sugar in the urine, frequent urination, and increase thirst" (American Diabetes Association, 2017c, p.1). Glucometers vary in brands and styles but generally operates in the same manner. Professional nurses/certified nursing assistants CENA's are generally familiar with these devices and may know how to operate and calibrate them. If not used correctly, the glucometer will also give false readings. In addition to assessing an individual's glucose (sugar) levels, if the individual is feeling short of breath the pulse oximeter may prove to be of value by measuring the individuals' oxygen level.

Pulse Oximeter

The pulse oximeter can be employed by professionals and non-professionals on nurses' guild. This device is placed on the individuals' finger and it measures "how much of the hemoglobin in blood is carrying oxygen (oxygen saturation) . . . Pulse oximeters are in common use because they are: non-invasive, cheap to buy and use, can be very compact, detects hypoxaemia earlier than you using your eyes to see cyanosis" (Word Press, 2012, p.1). Hypoxaemia is abnormal low levels of oxygen in blood (Mayo Clinic, 2017) and hemoglobin is the "protein molecule in red blood cells that carries oxygen from the lungs to the body's tissues and returns carbon dioxide from the tissues back to the lungs" (Davis, 2017, p.1). The pulse ox is generally taken on the index finger with the oximeter, and one should make sure the index fingernail is short.

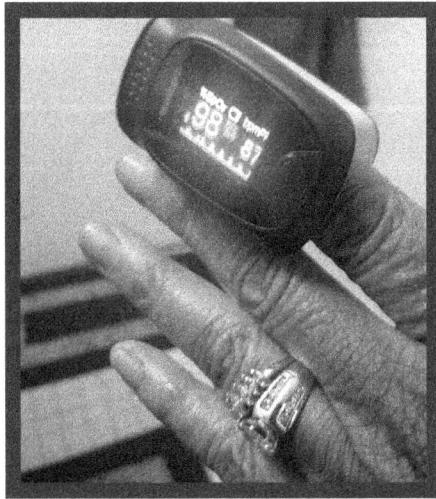

This device is easy and painless in measuring oxygen levels of the blood and detects how well the oxygen is sent to "parts of your body furthest from your heart, such as the arms and legs. A clip-like device called a probe is placed on a body part, such as a finger . . . Pulse oximetry is also used to check the health of a person with any condition that affects blood oxygen levels, such as: heart attack, chronic obstructive pulmonary disease (COPD), anemia, lung cancer, asthma, and pneumonia (John Hopkins Medicine, n.d.). Of course, when visiting your physicians pulse oximetry may be taken for other reasons. The normal range for pulse oximetry is 96-100 percent (Hoyle, 2017). Just as the oxygen levels change, many individuals temperature change. The nursing office being equipped with a thermometer is idea.

Thermometer

The thermometer measures the body's temperature. DiBenedetto (1993) expresses body temperature as an estimation of the average temperature of the core portions of the body as revealed by the temperature of the blood in the major vessels. The University of Michigan (2017) states a more plausible understanding of temperature:

> Body temperature is a measure of your body's ability to make and get rid of heat. The body is very good at keeping its temperature within a safe range, even when temperatures outside the body change a lot. When you are too hot, the blood vessels in your skin widen to carry the excess heat to your skin's surface. You may start to sweat. As the sweat evaporates, it helps cool your body. When you are too cold, your blood vessels narrow. This reduces blood flow to your skin to save body heat. You may start to shiver. When the muscles tremble this way, it helps to make more heat (p.1).

The normal body temperature is 98.6°F/37°C *(°F represents Fahrenheit and °C represents Celsius)*, yet there are many reasons why individuals temperature changes. Medline Plus (2017) posits:

Normal body temperature varies by person, age, activity, and time of day. The average normal body temperature is generally accepted as 98.6°F (37°C). Some studies have shown that the "normal" body temperature can have a wide range, from 97°F (36.1°C) to 99°F (37.2°C). A temperature over 100.4°F (38°C) most often means you have a fever caused by an infection or illness. Body temperature normally changes throughout the day (p.1).

While assessing one's temperature is idea in the projection of a fever, it is important as to what type of thermometer is being used.

The Danger of Using Mercury Thermometers

The temperature can be taken with several types of thermometers. The use of a digital or electronic thermometer is highly recommended. Never use a mercury thermometer which is highly toxic if broken. According to Thermometer Guide (2017):

The small silvery ball in a mercury thermometer can be dangerous if the glass breaks and the mercury is not cleaned up properly. The mercury will evaporate and can contaminate the surrounding air and become toxic to you and your family. Occasionally serious illness and even death results may occur from exposure to mercury from fever thermometers. However, if the consumer fails to clean up mercury either because he or she is unaware that it has broken or because it is difficult to gain access to the mercury (for instance because it has seeped through a carpet), then the mercury will/might reach dangerous levels in indoor air. The risks increase if the consumer attempts to clean up a mercury spill with a vacuum cleaner, or if the mercury is heated for some reason. The danger of significant mercury exposure is greatest in a small, poorly-ventilated room. Never use a vacuum cleaner as they do not pick up the drops and vacuuming vaporizes the mercury. Never use a broom as this breaks up the mercury further. Never pour it down the drain as this blocks the sink and harms the waterways. Never wash clothing with mercury spills on it as this will contaminate the washing machine and spread it, dispose of such clothing. To prevent possible contamination, stop using your mercury thermometer. Get a new, safer type of thermometer (p.1).

Some thermometers available to the public that accurately and expediently takes temperatures are: thermoscan ear thermometers, forehead thermometers, and digital thermometers which takes oral, rectal, and axillary (underarm) temperatures. Anyone can be trained to take temperatures. A key factor in taking an accurate oral temperature is to wait 5 minutes before taking the temperature if the individual has just consumed a hot or cold beverage. *FYI: The most accurate temperature is the rectal* temperature, second is oral temperature. Hot and cold packs may alter temperatures and proves to be of value in other emergency and non-emergency matters.

Hot/Cold Packs

Additional tools that may assist the church nurse in the event of emergency or non-emergency matters are hot and cold disposable packs. While one does not readily anticipate an injury, sometimes injuries happen. Hot and Cold packs are good therapy in the promotion of healing, decreasing inflammation, reducing joint and muscle pain, providing pain relief from minor injuries, muscle spasms, joint stiffness, and body aches. Yet there are precautions in applying hot and cold packs such as: *not applying them directly to the skin,* knowing *vital information about the individual* in need of the hot or cold pack, and *knowing when not to apply hot or cold packs.* Hot or Cold packs should never be applied "over areas of skin that are in poor condition, over areas of skin with poor sensation to heat or cold, over areas of the body with known poor circulation, if you have diabetes, or in the presence of infection" (Southern California Orthopedic Institute, n.d.).

As noted, having appropriate tools accessible for nurses on the guild will assist highly in attending to parishioners' needs. Still one must have knowledge as to why the appropriate tools are necessary, how to employ them, and most importantly the conditions of the individual to whom the service is being rendered. For the most part, some parishioners will not disclose valuable information to church nurses (professional or not) due to the fear of embarrassment or the feeling that it is not important. For example, one may ask the church nurse to take their blood pressure but will not disclose pertinent information regarding their blood pressure (the individual has a history of high blood pressure and are non-compliant in taking their prescribed blood pressure medications).

No worries, everyone has a right to refuse; after taking the blood pressure let the individual know the findings and refer them to the appropriate authorities i.e., emergency or their primary physician. Always remember to document your findings/referrals and the individuals' comments in log book kept under lock and key (in the nursing office). The church nurse should always ask questions from individuals asking for services rendered such as blood pressure, blood sugars and pulse oximetry readings, injuries requiring dressings, and CPR emergencies. Just as professional nursing, church nursing can be challenging but rewarding. As Christian church nurses we should accommodate our brothers and sisters in all matters possible; especially handicap parishioners that are in need of assistance.

Handicap Accommodations

How blessed it is to have a nurses' guild willing and ready to accommodate the pastor and other parishioners in any way possible, especially those who are handicapped and may have to use walkers, wheelchairs, canes, etc; for this very reason, churches equipped with handicap masonry ramps are highly welcoming. Some parishioners do not come to church because they feel it is too much of a fuss dealing with their wheelchairs or other devices entering in and out of the building. Handicap ramps are also beneficial in the event of an emergency in allowing easy access to the individual and if needed; transporting individuals out of the facility via car or the Emergency Medical Service (EMS).

Churches having the listed equipment can enhance the nurse' guild; the nurses should keep all equipment clean, and make sure all apparatuses needing batteries are changed frequently and tested for accuracy. If at all possible, there should be two of all vital equipments: blood pressure, glucometer, pulse ox, and temperature apparatuses available at the site along with extra batteries, since most of these apparatus use them. While individuals attend church with hopes of an uneventful ordeal, sometimes mishaps occur. In a society as today, one must expect the unexpected and be ready to react. Emergencies can be mindboggling and challenging, especially in the event of a heart attack. Even the most trained health professional can become nervous and forget the CPR protocol. Still when protocols are remembered, time is the most important essence. This brings us to the last, but most rewarding tool that can be beneficial to any organization. If at all possible, the nurses' office should be equipped with an automatic external defibrillator (AED). Although AED's are expensive, the nurses' guild can implement fundraisers to offset the cost. So what is an automatic external defibrillator and its significance? Duehring (2014) find:

> An AED is a computerized medical device that analyzes a person's heart rhythm, determines whether a shock is needed, and delivers a defibrillating shock if necessary. Owing to advances in technology, AEDs have become widely available and are safer, lighter, more portable, and easier to use than ever before. The prices of AEDs have also dropped significantly over the years. In the past, an AED could cost as much as $10,000, but these days, you can get an AED for around $1,500-$2,000. Most cardiac arrests are caused by ventricular fibrillation, an abnormal heart rhythm in which the heart flutters or quivers instead of pumping. The only recognized treatment for sudden cardiac arrest is early defibrillation, which shocks the heart back into a normal rhythm so that it can pump blood. The heart will not permit adequate circulation after

sudden cardiac arrest, even if CPR is performed. Using an AED immediately after sudden cardiac arrest can increase the chance of survival by more than 90%. The survival rate is reduced by approximately 10% for each minute that defibrillation is delayed. Placing an AED in your workplace can enhance employee morale, boost productivity, and improve employee safety and security (p.1).

I challenge AED's are not only beneficial in workplaces, but can benefit any organization in the event of an emergency. In addition to caring for the clergy and parishioners in one's assembly, the nurse's guild can sponsor or partnership with other organizations in efforts to assist individuals and families in their community.

Serving the Community

Nurses on the guild in assisting individuals and families in their community can sponsor minor and major events which incorporate selective planning. As my brother often posit, "When you fail to plan, you plan to fail" (Pastor Dr. Demetrius E. Ford, Ph.D., J.D., PsyD.). Every event should be planned effectively and in ample timeframes. One event the nurses' guild can sponsor that will benefit individuals in the community is a health fair which could only include informing individuals about their health (professional nurses and informational pamphlets available), taking blood pressure, and blood sugars levels. What about a food and clothing drive to service individuals in your church and community (some churches benefit from government grants to assist with these drives) who are in need of food and clothing?

With the high cost of living and few resources available in our society, people are greatly in need; yes, poverty exists everywhere, why not reach out and help someone. The Word of God confirms (paraphrased) that the poor will always be amongst us (Matthew 26:11; Mark 14:7), so let us love and assist one another. Often there are needy parishioners in our own church homes; yet they may be too proud to let others know. Let us as Christian nurses be diligent and humble in assessing and assisting our brother and sisters in Christ. One does not have to be a professional nurse to assist individuals in the church and the community in these manners. If the nurses' guild is unable to sponsor a drive, why not partnership with other organizations that sponsor drives (the American

Red Cross, hospitals, and others) in your community to assist individuals and families in need with events such as blood drives, mammogram screenings, prostate screenings, cholesterol, etc.

We as Christians (in representing the sheep of Christ) have a great responsibility in serving all mankind with love, kindness, and services; for we want our Lord to welcome us when we come into His Kingdom. Jesus states in Matthew 25: 34-36(NKJV), "Come, you blessed of My Father, inherit the kingdom prepared for you from the foundation of the world: for I was hungry and you gave Me food; I was thirsty and you gave Me drink; I was a stranger and you took Me in; I *was* naked and you clothed Me; I was sick and you visited Me; I was in prison and you came to Me. Jesus goes on to say in Matthew 25: 45(NKJV) . . . "Assuredly, I say to you, inasmuch as you did *it* to one of the least of these My brethren, you did *it* to Me."

It is a known fact that "He that hath pity upon the poor lendeth unto the LORD; and that which he hath given will He pay him again" (Proverbs 19:17). Dear Christian nurses on the guild, ". . . Let us not love in word, neither in tongue; but in deed and in truth." (1ˢᵗ John 3:18). Let us build up and assist one another. Let us flourish each other with brotherly love, and let us train our nurses to serve with pride and dignity in implementing all works for the Glory of God and the edification of mankind. As individuals and as a nurses' guild, we must continue to pray that God strengthens, unite our church families, biological families, our communities, and our nation. Let us remain steadfast in studying the Word of God for wisdom, knowledge, understanding, and strength while continuing to render service on our nurses' guilds. Non-medical personnel nurses on the guild (may be strengthened) in learning CPR may decrease some anxiety while responding to medical emergencies. In addition, individuals on the nurses' guild or perhaps a parishioner (one does not have to be in the medical field to apply) can choose to teach others by becoming certified to teach the CPR course. Listed below is information in regards to becoming a CPR Certified Instructor.

CHAPTER 7
HOW TO BECOME A CPR CERTIFIED INSTRUCTOR

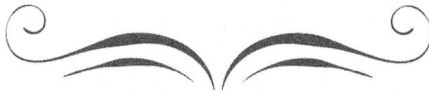

Overall, the nurses' guild members are typically responsible for serving the church' pulpit staff and often the first responders to persons who may faint or suffer other moments of physical distress in church. As with professional nurses, more and more church nurses are becoming certified in First Aid and CPR as an added benefit to the auxiliary and parishioners. All members on the guild should be willing to obtain first aid and cardiopulmonary resuscitation (CPR) certification; yet in my humble opinion CPR should not be mandated, especially if an elderly or youth individual desire to join the guild. Even without CPR, individuals can be trained to *expect* the *unexpected* and *be ready to respond to any life threatening emergency*.

Again, the qualifications and duties of a church nurse vary from one organization to another. Churches equipped with medical professionals on their nurse' guild may give parishioners a great since of comfort just knowing they are readily accessible on their guild. Overall, many Baptist churches are requiring members of the nurses' guild to be certified in First aid and CPR. Interesting, while conducting research on church nursing, one church nurses' guild qualifications caught my eye in being proactive in preparing for medical emergencies. The statement read, the qualifications of a church nurse should include: nurses as being saved, willing to serve, trained and certified in cardiopulmonary resuscitation, first aid, automatic external defibrillator (AED) maintained up-to-date, and should include professionals such as registered nurses (RN's), licensed practical nurses (LPN's), medical assistances (MA's), certified nurse aids (CNA's), and they must be committed (National Baptist Convention, 2014).

Again, I agree that First Aid and CPR certification should be offered and recommended; but not mandated. I contend that anyone willing to serve on the nurses' guild should be permitted to join and willing to enhance their skills if feasible for the individual. Some individual are unable to perform the

CPR tasks but desire to be a church nurse and should not be turned away in rendering services to the Lord. In my modest opinion, *church nursing* is not to be compared with *professional nursing.* As church nursing operated sufficiently in the days of old, it still will operate sufficiently now. *Give me that old time religion; what did we do back in the day?* For the most part, some people become very nervous in the event of an emergency (even professional nurses) and may perform emergency tasks incorrectly. This does not mean that they will not make a good church nurse; I recommend allowing them to join the guild and leave the professional tasks for the nurses that have medical credentials and certifications. While the unlicensed church nurse may not be able to perform emergency tasks, they certainly can perform other tasks in serving the clergy/parishioners and perform other non-emergency duties if trained by professional health personnel. Some churches hire professional personnel to come in and train the nurses on the guild in first-aid and CPR, now this measure I certainly agree with.

Some church nursing guilds may be fortunate to have a CPR certified instructor on the guild or in the congregation. If not, the course is readily available to anyone who meets the minimum requirements and desires to become a CPR certified instructor. The pay is good (average of $43,840 annually) and the training is rewarding in knowing that you assist others in learning the vital steps that may save a person's life. The requirements are listed below and for the most part, only a high school diploma is required in addition to other minor details. Some facts to consider before deciding to become a Certified CPR Instructor are: CPR Duties: coordinating class times and locations, transporting and cleaning equipment, evaluating students performance and ensuring completion of required paperwork, and lifting of heavy equipment (mannequins).

Meeting the Requirements for the CPR Instructor

Requirements to obtain certification as a basic life support instructor are reasonable. One needs only to obtain a high school diploma and a certification in Basic Life Support as well as 2-3 years of teaching as a Basic Life certified instructor (sometimes required). Various organizations such as the American Red Cross (ARC), American Heart Association (AHA), National Safety Council and the American Safety and Health Institute offer courses for healthcare providers and non-healthcare providers who require (Study.com, 2016) or desire certification. If one is working in a health care environment, please check with your employer to see if a Basic Life Support certified CPR Course is offered at your facility at no cost to you as an employee. You must be able to lift at least 50 pounds and able to perform CPR, have a valid driver's license, and possess good customer service skills, speaking, teaching, and presentations skills.   The individual must also be computer orientated and have knowledge of Microsoft Office suite (Study.com, 2016).

The candidate for the CPR instructor must contact the American Heart Association after obtaining their certification in Basic Life Support to assure they are accepting new instructors (this is a requirement). *There is no pre-course exam for training at the AHA*; however if one plan to train at the ARC, they must register for the initial pre-course exam and pass this exam which is a prerequisite to attending the instructor course which is offered by the Red Cross (Study.com, 2016).

Instructor Requirements at the Red Cross

The instructor training courses offered by the American Red Cross (ARC) consist of two courses. *The first course at the*

ARC consists of series and is called Fundamentals of Instructor Training (FIT). This course introduces the students to the ARC organization and consists of the history, activities, and the organizational structure. The majority ARC instructor courses are designed for a specific audience and prepare instructors to work with that specific audience after completion (Study.com, 2016). Many classes are offered online, in a classroom and in mixture formats. The ARC instructor certifications are valid for two years and may be renewed with minimum requirements (instructor taught at least one CPR course) as long as it is within the certification period (Study.com, 2016).

Instructor Requirements at the American Heart Association

The instructor training courses offered by the AHA also consist of two courses. The *first instructor course at the AHA* is called the Core Instructor Course which teaches planning and preparation, methods of instruction, management, assessment and cultural sensitivity through a series of 20 interactive training modules (Study.com, 2016). This course is offered online, in a classroom, or via a compact disc (CD) in a self-directed format. Upon successful completion of this course, the student is given a certificate. AHA instructor's courses train the prospective student in CPR, Basic Life Support, Heartsaver, Advanced Cardiac Life Support and Pediatric Advanced Life Support. The new AHA instructor will be monitored while teaching their first class in fulfilling the course requirement; this is not a requirement for the ARC. All AHA instructors are required to teach at least four classes during the two-year certification period. AHA-certified instructors must pass a re-certify exam (Study.com, 2016). For both the ARC and the AHA, one can access their online networks for more information regarding becoming a CPR instructor. After signing up and becoming an instructor one will have full access to training materials, manage your course records, print certificates and more (Study.com, 2016).

CONCLUSIONS

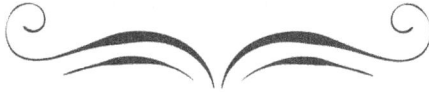

Nurse's guilds in the Baptist church have existed for decades and each year one denotes trends. This book is intended as a template for those who need just a little guidance. While all the information may not be employed, it really is something to contemplate on in strengthening your guild. Implementing a nurses' guild or any new auxiliary in the church (small, medium, or large church) can be challenging but rewarding. One main challenge is finding dedicated individuals who love the Lord and really want to render services to Him. While many interventions will be trial and error, one must determine what works best for their assembly.

Trials and errors teach one to become prudent and proactive in the prevention of errors. Some salient point learned over my past years as a church nurse includes; knowing the preferences of my pastor and other ministers on the rostrum such as their preferred beverages, how they prefer their beverages to be served (some prefer cold with ice, while others prefer room temperature or hot), and what they prefer to use when wiping their faces. Some ministers prefer handkerchiefs, while others prefer towels after speaking or preaching. Other preference included knowing how to assist my pastor and other clergy in relationship to having necessary items available after they preach, and knowing when and where to serve them.

Some ministers become engulfed with sweat while delivering the message and prefer to change their shirt (in the pastor' study), put on a cape, or perhaps their coat (while in the pulpit). I also learned the significance of respecting the areas in the church in which nurses are allowed to enter and serve. It is very important to know where nurses are allowed to serve ministers in the church; some churches allow their nurses to serve in the pulpit while other does not. All questions should be asked prior to joining a nurses' guild and prior to the start of service in which the assigned nurse are to serve. Nurses in being prudent should arrive early on the day assigned to serve to inquire from clergy their preferences while they are in the office. Always prepare for the unexpected (as in bringing or keeping extra materials) in anticipating what is needed prior to the start of service.

While there may be five ministers present on the rostrum, only one may want service; and vice versa. Yes, this has happened to me, in fact there were seven which desired services, and being proactive in bringing extras all were served, praise God. Always expect the unexpected, serve with kindness and sincerity, in the name of the Lord; for greater is your reward in heaven. Nurses on the guild should be prudent and proactive in asserting equipment is working properly with batteries changed frequently. Always check and maintain good functioning vital equipment such as blood pressure, glucometers, and pulse ox machines.

I pray that this book is helpful, inspiring, and edifying to all who serve or desire to serve on nurse's guilds all around the world. I thank God for allowing me to be His servant in serving on the nurses' guild, for He knows I love Him and nursing; it's not surprising that I chose nursing as my profession and many others have also. Just as nurses are in demand for the nurse's guild in churches, nurses are in demand as a profession. Perhaps you should consider becoming a professional nurse as well as serving on your church's nurses' guild, both are rewarding. FYI: Nursing is the fastest-growing occupation in the US and make up the majority of the healthcare industry and that number is going up, with 581,300 more nursing jobs by 2018. Why? There are a lot of reasons, including an aging population and a shrinking nursing workforce (Johnson & Johnson, 2017). According to Every Nurse.org (n.d.):

> As one of the fastest growing occupations in the U.S., there is a greater need in the nation (and across the world) to hire nurses than any other healthcare worker in the industry. According to Deborah D'Avolio, PhD, ACNP, ANP, an Associate Professor at Northeastern University's Bouve College of Health Sciences School of Nursing, "a nurse is an expert clinician, scientist, healer, health translator, communicator, teacher, guide, and family supporter" – all of which are needed to ensure the health and wellness of individuals, families, and communities (p. 1).

Are you ready to come on board? "God is not unjust, He will not forget your work and the love you have shown Him as you helped His people and continue to help them" (Hebrew 6:10). Why not pledge to become a church or professional nurse; *the Florence Nightingale Pledge although, emulated by*

professional nurses can be employed in church nursing as well.
God Bless!

1935 Revised Version of the Florence Nightingale Pledge

I solemnly pledge myself before God and in the presence of this assembly to pass my life in purity and to practice my profession faithfully. I will abstain from whatever is deleterious and mischievous, and will not take or knowingly administer any harmful drug. I will do all in my power to maintain and elevate the standard of my profession and will hold in confidence all personal matters committed to my keeping and all family affairs coming to my knowledge in the practice of my calling. With loyalty will I aid the physician in his work, and as a missioner of health, I will dedicate myself to devoted service for human welfare (Wikipedia, 2016c).

REFERENCES

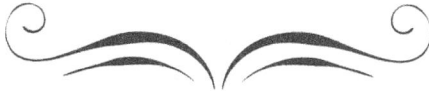

American College of Allergy, Asthma, & Immunology (2014). Latex allergy. *ACAAI.* Retrieved from http://acaai.org/allergies/types/skin-allergies/latex-allergy

American Diabetes Association (2017a). Checking your blood glucose. *ADA.* Retrieved from http://www.diabetes.org/living-with-diabetes/treatment-and-care/blood-glucose-control/checking-your-blood-glucose.html

American Diabetes Association (2017b). Hypoglycemia (low blood glucose). *ADA.* Retrieved from http://www.diabetes.org/living-with-diabetes/treatment-and-care/blood-glucose-control/hypoglycemia-low-blood.html

American Diabetes Association (2017c). Hyperglycemia (high blood glucose). *ADA.* Retrieved from http://www.diabetes.org/living-with-diabetes/treatment-and-care/blood-glucose-control/hyperglycemia.html

American Heart Association (2017).   Understanding blood pressure

readings. *AHA*. Retrieved from

http://www.heart.org/HEARTORG/Conditions/HighBloodPr

essure/KnowYourNumbers/Understanding-Blood-Pressure-

Readings_UCM_301764_Article.jsp#.WeUyFr3mtcM

American Nurses Association. (2016). What is nursing?

Nursingworld.org. Retrieved from

http://www.nursingworld.org/EspeciallyForYou/What-is-

Nursing

Ansell. (2017).   Know the difference: Why non-latex gloves.

Gammax. Retrieved from http://www.ansell.com/en-

US/Campaigns/Non-Latex-Conversion/Why-Non-

Latex/Why-Non-Latex.aspx

Bible Study Tools. (2016). *Deacon, deaconess.* Retrieved from

http://www.biblestudytools.com/dictionaries/bakers-

evangelical-dictionary/deacon-deaconess.html

Davis, C. P. (2017).   What is Hemoglobin? *Medicine Net.* Retrieved

from

https://www.medicinenet.com/hemoglobin/article.htm

DiBenedetto, L. (1993).   Core Temperature. *IVAC Corporation*: San

Diego, CA.

Discovernursing.com.   *Why be a nurse?* Retrieved from

https://www.discovernursing.com/why-be-a-

nurse#.WBywfb3mvDw

Duehring, S. (June, 2014). AED program in the Workplace: Benefits of implementing an AED program in the workplace. *EMC CPR & Safety Training*. Retrieved from http://www.emccprtraining.com/blog/emc-news-and-updates/workplace-cpr-aed/benefits-of-implementing-an-aed-program-in-the-workplace

Early, J. (January, 2016). Nursing cap collection. *Museum of Nursing History*. Retrieved from http://www.nursinghistory.org/nursing-cap-collection/

Evers, M. (2012). The *African American lectionary: Cultural resources*. Retrieved from http://www.theafricanamericanlectionary.org/PopupCulturalAid.asp?LRID=411

Every Nurse.org (n.d.). *Why nursing?* Retrieved from: http://everynurse.org/become-nurse/

Farlex (2017). Fomite. *The Free Dictionary*. Retrieved from http://medical-dictionary.thefreedictionary.com/f

Google.com. (n.d.). Nurse. *Google.* Retrieved from https://www.google.com/?gws_rd=ssl#q=what+is+a+nurse

Greater Progressive Baptist Church (2012). *Nurses ministry*. Retrieved from http://www.greaterprogressive.org/nurses-ministry/

Hoyle, G. M. (2017). Normal pulse oximetry. *Livestrong.com*.

Retrieved from
https://www.livestrong.com/article/244285-
disadvantages-of-pulse-oximetry/

John Hopkins Medicine (n.d.). Pulse oximetry. *The John Hopkins
University*. Retrieved from
http://www.hopkinsmedicine.org/healthlibrary/test_proce
dures/pulmonary/oximetry_92,p07754

Laity Services Committee. (n.d.). *Laity Services Committee of the
Lutheran Deaconess Association*. Retrieved from
http://www.thelda.org/assets/docs/history_deacs_nurses.
pdf

Mayo Clinic (2017). Hypoxemia (low blood oxygen*). Mayo
Foundation for Medical Education and Research (MFMER)*.
Retrieved from
https://www.mayoclinic.org/symptoms/hypoxemia/basics/
definition/SYM-20050930

Medline Plus. (October, 2017). Body temperature norms.
Medlineplus.gov. Retrieved from
https://medlineplus.gov/ency/article/001982.htm

Nurses Service Organization (2017). Administer meds without a
doctor's order? Proceed with caution. *Affinity Insurance
Services*. Retrieved from http://www.nso.com/risk-
education/individuals/articles/Administer-Meds-Without-
a-Doctors-Order-Proceed-With-Caution

Jaret, P. (2017). Fainting and loss of consciousness. *Health day: News for healthier living.* Retrieved from https://consumer.healthday.com/encyclopedia/first-aid-and-emergencies-20/emergencies-and-first-aid-news-227/fainting-and-loss-of-consciousness-644511.html

Johnson & Johnson. (2017). *Why be a nurse?* Retrieved from: https://www.discovernursing.com/why-be-a-nurse#.Wduoeb3mtcM

Lueders-Bolwerk, C. A. (January, 2009). What is parish nursing? *NSNA Imprint.* Retrieved from http://www.nsna.org/Portals/0/Skins/NSNA/pdf/Imprint_J an09_Feat_Lueders.pdf

Merriam-Webster. (2016). Full definition of nurse. *Merriam-Webster .com.* Retrieved from http://www.merriam-Webster.com/dictionary/nurse

Merriam-Webster. (n.d.). Deaconess. *Merriam-Webster.com.* Retrieved from http://www.merriam-webster.com/dictionary/deaconess

National Baptist Convention (2014). *Ushers and nurses auxiliary: Ushers and nurses 2014 annual session.* Retrieved from http://resources.razorplanet.com/510611-8783/1086527_ChurchNursesDutiesQualifications.pdf

Neff, S. (n.d.). Parish nurse. *The English district of the Lutheran church-Missouri synod.* Retrieved from http://www.englishdistrict.org/ministries/parish-nurse

Savva, G. (May, 2017). Anxiety and fear of the unknown: Anxiety, stress, and panic. *Counselling Directory*. Retrieved from http://www.counselling-directory.org.uk/counsellor-articles/anxiety-and-fear-of-the-unknown

Soares, C. (October, 2015). Latex allergy awareness week: Understanding the dangers of latex overexposure. *Medic Alert*. Retrieved from https://www.medicalert.org/Latex_Allergy_%20Awareness_Week%202015

Southern California Orthopedic Institute (n.d.). Should you ice or heat an injury? *SCOI*. Retrieved from https://www.scoi.com/patient-resources/health-articles/should-you-ice-or-heat-injury

Study.com. (2016). *How to become a certified CPR instructor*. Retrieved from http://study.com/articles/How_to_Become_a_Certified_CPR_Instructor.html

The Bible Study Site (n.d.). *Meaning of the color white in the Bible*. Retrieved from http://www.biblestudy.org/bible-study-by-topic/meaning-of-colors-in-the-bible/meaning-of-color-white.html

The Holy Bible. (2011). New International Version (NIV). *Biblica Incorporation*. Retrieved from

https://www.biblegateway.com/passage/?search=Romans
%2015:1-7

The Holy Bible. (1998). King James Version (KJV). Large print
compact edition. *Holman Bible Publishers:* Korea.

Thermometer Guide. (n.d.). The dangers of mercury
thermometers. *Thermomerterguide.com.* Retrieved from
http://www.thermometerguide.com/the-dangers-of-
mercury-thermometers/

The Truth About Nursing. (2002). What is nursing?
Thetruthaboutnursing.org. Retrieved from
http://www.truthaboutnursing.org/faq/nursing_definition.
html

Thunderwolf. (2006). Men in nursing: A historical time line.
Allnurses.com. Retrieved from http://allnurses.com/men-
in-nursing/men-in-nursing-96326.html

University of Michigan. (2017). Body temperature: Test overview.
Michigan Medicine University of Michigan. Retrieved from
http://www.uofmhealth.org/health-library/hw198785

U.S. Census Bureau. (February, 2013). *Men in nursing occupations:
American community surveys highlight report.* Retrieved
from
https://www.census.gov/people/io/files/Men_in_Nursing_

Occupations.pdf

Webster Dictionary (1913). *White.* Retrieved from
http://www.webster-dictionary.org/definition/white

Wikipedia. (October, 2017). White. *Wikipedia the Free
Encyclopedia.* Retrieved from
https://en.wikipedia.org/wiki/White

Wikipedia. (October, 2016a). Smelling salts. *Wikipedia the Free
Encyclopedia.* Retrieved from
https://en.wikipedia.org/wiki/Smelling_salts

Wikipedia. (October, 2016b). Florence Nightingale. *Wikipedia the
Free Encyclopedia.* Retrieved from
https://en.wikipedia.org/wiki/Florence_Nightingale

Wikipedia. (October, 2016c). Nightingale pledge. *Wikipedia the
Free Encyclopedia.* Retrieved from
https://en.wikipedia.org/wiki/Nightingale_Pledge

Wikipedia. (October, 2016d). Nurse uniform. *Wikipedia the Free
Encyclopedia.* Retrieved from
https://en.wikipedia.org/wiki/Nurse_uniform

Wikipedia. (November, 2016). Deaconess. *Wikipedia, the Free
Encyclopedia.* Retrieved from
https://en.wikipedia.org/wiki/Deaconess

Word Press (2012). Oxygen saturation. *Howequipmentwork.com*.

Retrieved from

https://www.howequipmentworks.com/pulse_oximeter/

ABOUT
THE AUTHOR

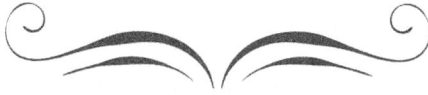

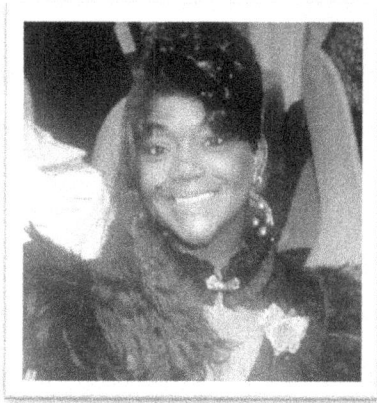

Dr. Juanita Crawford has been a church nurse for over 30 years and a professional nurse for 27.5 years. Her background includes: Medical- Surgical Staff Nurse, Charge Nurse, Interim Clinic Nurse Manager, Nursing Mentor, Telephone Triage Nurse, and an Ambulatory Care Nurse in various areas: Pediatrics, Obstetrics (OB), Gynecology (GYN), Orthopedics, Internal Medicine, Podiatry, and Surgical Outpatient. Dr. Crawford currently works as an Adjunct Nursing Professor (14 years) with Registered Nursing students

(RN's) and (3 years) with Licensed Practical Nursing students (LPN's). She has been singing since the age of five as a Gospel Soloist, and enjoys being a Church Nurse, Nursing Professor, and Housewife. Her Doctorate Degree is in Education and her Master's Degree is in Nursing. Hobbies (Unprofessionally includes): Cosmetology, Barber, and Seamstress. Other Hobbies includes: Singing, Reading, Writing, Arts and Crafts; but most importantly spending quality time with family and friends.

WITH GOD ALL THINGS ARE POSSIBLE